BARIATRIC DIET COOKBOOK

A Complete guide to long-term wellness with Tasty, delicious & Nutritious healthy recipes…

BY

Mildred Kent

TABLE OF CONTENT

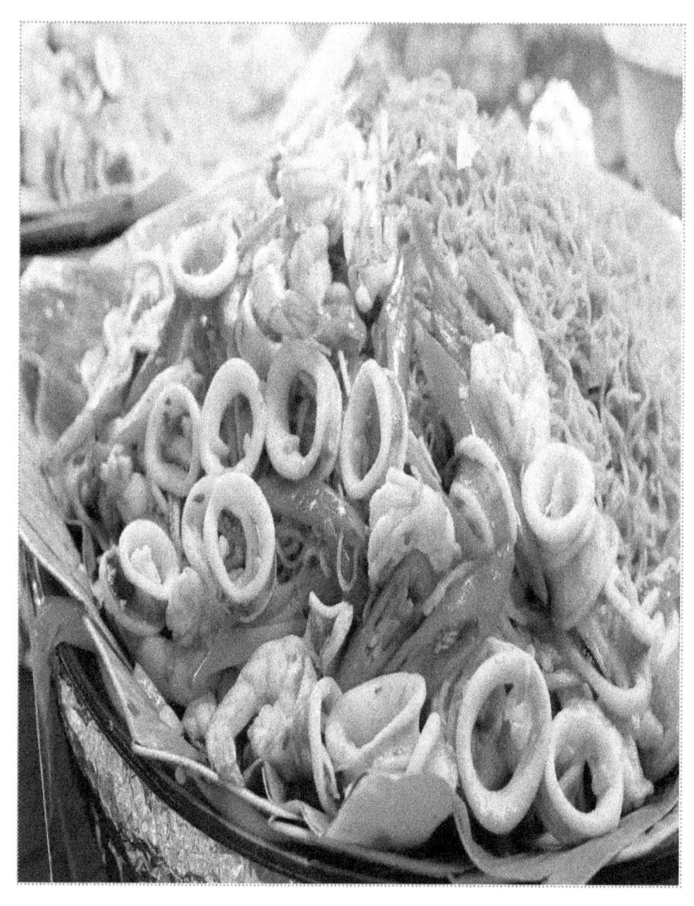

CHAPTER ONE

1. SARAH SHORT STORY

Sarah sat in her doctor's office, her heart pounding with a mix of hope and anxiety. For years, she had struggled with her weight, trying every diet and exercise plan under the sun without success. But now, her doctor was suggesting something different: "bariatric surgery"…

1.2 Introduction to Bariatric Surgery

Bariatric surgery is a life-changing procedure designed to help individuals who are severely overweight or obese achieve significant weight loss. It's not a decision to be taken lightly, but for many people like Sarah, it offers a new beginning—a chance to break free from the cycle of obesity and reclaim their health.

There are several different types of bariatric surgery, but they all work by either restricting the amount of food the stomach can hold, reducing the body's ability to absorb nutrients, or a combination of both. Some of the most common procedures include gastric bypass, sleeve gastrectomy, and adjustable gastric banding.

1.3 Overview of Bariatric Surgery

Gastric bypass surgery, often considered the gold standard of bariatric procedures, involves creating a small pouch at the top of the stomach and rerouting the intestines to bypass a portion of the digestive tract. This not only reduces the amount of food a person can eat at one time but also alters the way their body absorbs calories.

Sleeve gastrectomy, on the other hand, involves removing a large portion of the stomach to create a smaller, banana-shaped pouch. This restricts the amount of food that can be consumed and also reduces the production of hunger-inducing hormones, helping patients feel full faster and stay satisfied longer.

Adjustable gastric banding is a less invasive option that involves placing a silicone band around the upper part of the stomach, creating a small pouch and a narrow passage into the rest of the stomach. The band can be adjusted to control the size of the opening, allowing for customized weight loss.

Regardless of the specific procedure, bariatric surgery is intended to jump-start weight loss and improve overall health. But it's important to remember that surgery is just the beginning of the journey—not the end.

1.4 Importance of Diet Post-Surgery

After bariatric surgery, patients must commit to making significant lifestyle changes, particularly when it comes to their diet. This is because the surgery alters the way the body processes food, making it essential to follow a specific eating plan to ensure long-term success.

Immediately following surgery, patients are typically placed on a strict liquid diet to allow the stomach to heal. Over time, they gradually transition to soft foods and then eventually solid foods, with a focus on lean protein, fruits, vegetables, and whole grains.

Portion control is key, as the new, smaller stomach pouch can only hold a limited amount of food at once. Eating too much or too quickly can lead to discomfort, nausea, and vomiting, so it's important for patients to listen to their bodies and stop eating when they feel full.

In addition to watching what they eat, patients must also pay attention to how they eat. Chewing food thoroughly, eating slowly, and avoiding drinking liquids with meals can help prevent complications and maximize weight loss results.

But perhaps most importantly, bariatric surgery patients must be committed to making lasting changes to their eating habits and lifestyle.

Surgery is a powerful tool, but it's not a magic bullet. Success requires dedication, discipline, and a willingness to embrace a new way of living.

For Sarah, bariatric surgery was the beginning of a new chapter in her life. It wasn't always easy, but with the support of her medical team and the determination to stick to her post-surgery diet, she gradually began to see the pounds melt away and her health improve.

Today, Sarah is happier and healthier than she's been in years. Bariatric surgery may have given her the push she needed to start her weight loss journey, but it was her commitment to following a healthy diet and making positive lifestyle changes that ultimately led to her success.

CHAPTER TWO

2.   Understanding the Bariatric Diet

Bariatric surgery can be a life-changing procedure for those struggling with severe obesity. But it's not just about the surgery itself; it's also about adopting a whole new lifestyle, including a specific diet. Understanding the bariatric diet is crucial for successful weight loss and long-term health.

2.1   Principles of the Bariatric Diet

The bariatric diet isn't a one-size-fits-all plan. It's tailored to the individual needs of each patient based on the type of surgery they've had (such as gastric bypass or gastric sleeve) and their specific health goals. However, there are some general principles that apply to most bariatric diets.

Firstly, protein is king. After surgery, the stomach is much smaller, which means there's less room for food. Protein is essential for maintaining muscle mass and promoting healing, so it's prioritized in the diet. Good sources of protein include fish, poultry, eggs, and dairy products.

Next up, hydration is key. Drinking enough water is essential for everyone, but it's especially crucial for bariatric patients. Since they can't consume large amounts of food at once, getting enough fluids is vital for preventing dehydration and promoting proper digestion.

Another principle is to focus on nutrient-dense foods. With a smaller stomach capacity, every bite counts. So, it's essential to choose foods that are rich in vitamins, minerals, and other essential nutrients. This means plenty of fruits, vegetables, whole grains, and healthy fats.

Portion control is also critical. Bariatric patients must relearn how to listen to their bodies' hunger and fullness cues since overeating can lead to discomfort and complications. Eating small, frequent meals throughout the day can help prevent this and keep energy levels stable.

Finally, the bariatric diet isn't just about what you eat—it's also about how you eat. Chewing food thoroughly, eating slowly, and avoiding distractions like TV or smartphones during meals can all help prevent overeating and promote proper digestion.

2.2   Dietary Guidelines and Restrictions

While the bariatric diet emphasizes protein, hydration, nutrient-dense foods, and portion control, there are also some foods and beverages that should be limited or avoided altogether.

One big no-no is sugary and high-calorie beverages like soda, fruit juice, and energy drinks. Not only do these drinks provide empty calories, but they can also contribute to dumping syndrome—a condition where food moves too quickly from the stomach to the small intestine, causing symptoms like nausea, vomiting, and diarrhea.

High-fat and high-sugar foods should also be limited. These can include things like fried foods, sweets, pastries, and fatty meats. Not only are these foods calorie-dense, but they can also be difficult to digest, leading to discomfort and potentially even more serious complications.

Alcohol is another substance that should be consumed in moderation, if at all. Not only does alcohol provide empty calories, but it can also be absorbed more quickly into the bloodstream after bariatric surgery, leading to increased intoxication and a higher risk of accidents or injuries.

It's also essential to avoid certain foods that can cause gastrointestinal discomfort or obstruction, such as tough meats, fibrous vegetables, and sticky foods like bread and rice. Instead, opt for softer, easier-to-digest options like tender meats, cooked vegetables, and well-cooked grains.

2.3   Portion Control and Meal Frequency

Portion control is a fundamental aspect of the bariatric diet. Since the stomach is significantly smaller after surgery, it's crucial to eat smaller meals to avoid discomfort and ensure proper digestion. This means measuring out serving sizes, using smaller plates and utensils, and avoiding second helpings.

Meal frequency is also essential. Instead of three large meals a day, bariatric patients often find it more comfortable to eat five or six smaller meals throughout the day. This helps prevent overeating, keeps energy levels stable, and promotes better digestion.

It's also essential to space out meals and snacks throughout the day, allowing the stomach enough time to digest food fully before the next meal. This can help prevent symptoms like nausea, vomiting, and discomfort, and promote better overall digestion and nutrient absorption.

In addition to portion control and meal frequency, it's also essential to pay attention to how you eat. Chewing food thoroughly, eating slowly, and taking small bites can all help prevent overeating and promote better digestion. Avoiding distractions like TV or smartphones during meals can also help you stay mindful of what and how much you're eating.

Lastly, the bariatric diet is about more than just what you eat—it's about adopting a whole new approach to food and eating. By focusing on protein, hydration, nutrient-dense foods, portion control, and meal frequency, bariatric patients can support their weight loss goals and enjoy better overall health and well-being.

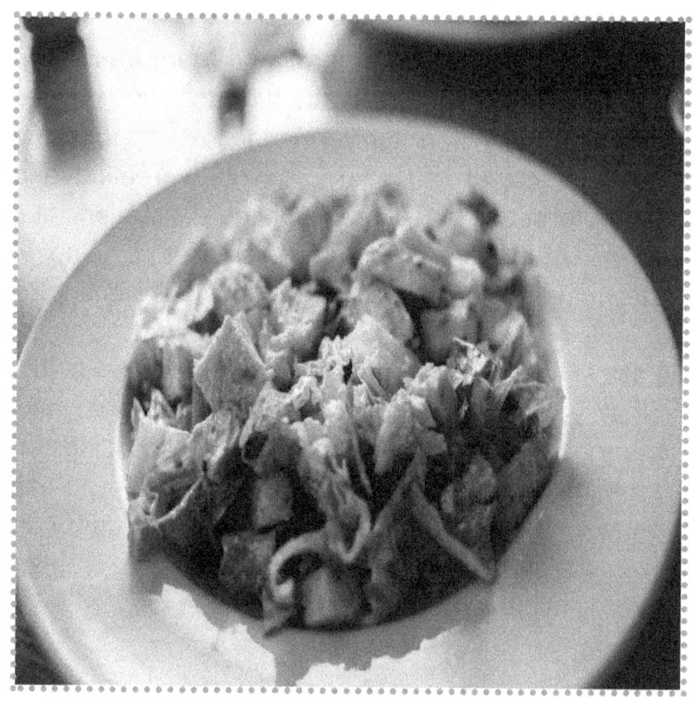

CHAPTER THREE

3. Preparing for Success

So, you're kick-starting on a journey toward healthier living through bariatric cooking. Congrats! But like any journey, preparation is key. How to position yourself for success is as follows:

First things first, educate yourself. Learn about bariatric cooking—what it entails, which foods are best suited, and how portion sizes differ post-surgery. How to position yourself for success is as follows:Knowing the fundamentals will provide you with a strong base from which to grow.

Next, clear out your kitchen. Say goodbye to tempting treats and processed foods that might derail your progress. Stock up instead on nutritious staples like lean proteins, veggies, fruits, and whole grains. Having the right ingredients on hand makes healthy cooking a breeze.

Now, let's talk about equipment. Invest in tools that make bariatric cooking easier, like a good set of knives, measuring cups, and a food scale. You'll also want to consider small appliances like a blender or food processor for pureeing foods to the right consistency.

3.1 Setting Realistic Goals

Setting realistic goals is crucial for success in any endeavor, including bariatric cooking. Here's how to do it:

Start by thinking about what you want to achieve. Maybe it's losing a certain amount of weight, improving your overall health, or simply feeling more comfortable in your own skin. Whatever your goals, make sure they're specific, measurable, and achievable.

After you've determined your objectives, divide them up into more manageable, smaller steps. For example, if your ultimate goal is to lose 50 pounds, set smaller milestones along the way, like losing 5 pounds in the first month.

Remember to be patient with yourself. Rome wasn't built in a day, and neither will your new healthy habits. Progress takes time, so celebrate your successes along the way, no matter how small.

3.2   Kitchen Essentials for Bariatric Cooking,

Now let's talk about the must-have items for your bariatric kitchen:

First up, a good set of knives. Sharp knives make chopping and prepping veggies a breeze, which is essential for bariatric cooking.

Next, invest in quality cookware. Look for pots and pans that distribute heat evenly to prevent burning and ensure that your meals cook evenly.

A food scale is another essential tool for bariatric cooking. It helps you accurately portion out your meals, which is crucial for post-surgery success.

Don't forget about storage containers! Having plenty of containers on hand makes it easy to portion out meals ahead of time and store leftovers for later.

And finally, consider investing in small appliances like a blender or food processor. These tools are great for pureeing foods to the right consistency, which is important for bariatric patients.

3.3 Meal Planning Tips under bariatric cooking,

Meal planning is key to staying on track with your bariatric diet. Here are some pointers to get you going:

Start by making a weekly meal plan. Sit down and decide what you're going to eat for breakfast, lunch, and dinner each day of the week. Don't forget to plan for snacks too!

Once you've planned your meals, make a shopping list and head to the grocery store. Stick to your list to avoid impulse buys and temptation.

When planning your meals, focus on protein-rich foods like lean meats, eggs, and tofu. Protein is essential for bariatric patients as it helps promote muscle growth and repair.

Don't forget about veggies! Aim to fill half your plate with non-starchy vegetables at each meal to help you feel full and satisfied.

CHAPTER FOUR

4. Bariatric-Friendly Recipes

Bariatric surgery is a life-changing procedure that requires a significant shift in eating habits. It's crucial to choose foods that are not only nutritious but also gentle on the stomach and promote weight loss. Here, we'll explore a variety of bariatric-friendly recipes tailored to different meals throughout the day.

4.1 Breakfast Options

1. Protein-Packed Smoothie:

- Start your day with a nutritious blend of protein powder, Greek yogurt, spinach, and a handful of berries. This smoothie provides essential nutrients without overloading your stomach.

2. Veggie Egg Muffins:

- Whip up a batch of mini egg muffins loaded with diced vegetables like bell peppers, onions, and spinach. These bite-sized delights are easy to prepare and can be stored for quick breakfasts during the week.

3. Overnight Oats:

- Combine rolled oats with Greek yogurt, almond milk, and your favorite fruits such as sliced bananas or berries. Let it sit overnight in the fridge, and in the morning, you'll have a satisfying and fiber-rich breakfast ready to enjoy.

4.2 Lunch and Dinner Recipes

1. Grilled Chicken Salad:

- Before grilling, marinate chicken breasts in a mixture of olive oil, lemon juice, and herbs. Serve sliced chicken over a bed of mixed greens, cherry tomatoes, cucumbers, and avocado for a filling yet light meal.

2. Zucchini Noodles with Turkey Meatballs:

- Swap traditional pasta for spiralized zucchini noodles and pair them with lean turkey meatballs. Top with marinara sauce and a sprinkle of Parmesan cheese for a guilt-free Italian-inspired dish.

3. Baked Salmon with Roasted Vegetables:

- Season salmon filets with herbs and a squeeze of lemon juice before baking in the oven. Roast a medley of vegetables like carrots, broccoli, and cauliflower alongside for a balanced and flavorful dinner.

4.3 Snacks and Appetizers

1. Greek Yogurt Dip with Veggies:

- Mix Greek yogurt with garlic powder, dill, and lemon juice to create a creamy dip. Serve with an assortment of fresh vegetables such as carrot sticks, cucumber slices, and bell pepper strips for a crunchy and satisfying snack.

2. Almond Butter Celery Sticks:

- Spread almond butter on celery sticks and top with a sprinkle of chia seeds for added crunch. This simple yet nutritious snack provides a satisfying combination of protein, fiber, and healthy fats.

3. Baked Sweet Potato Chips:

- Slice sweet potatoes thinly, toss with olive oil and seasonings, then bake until crispy. These homemade chips are a healthier alternative to store-bought snacks and can be enjoyed guilt-free.

4.4   Desserts and Treats

1. Berry Parfait:

- Layer Greek yogurt with mixed berries and a sprinkle of granola for a light and refreshing dessert option. This parfait is rich in antioxidants and satisfies your sweet cravings without excess sugar.

2. Chocolate Avocado Mousse:

- Blend ripe avocados with cocoa powder, honey, and a splash of almond milk until smooth and creamy. Chill in the refrigerator for a few hours to let the flavors meld together, then indulge in this decadent yet bariatric-friendly treat.

3. Frozen Banana Bites:

- Cut bananas into rounds, coat them with melted dark chocolate, and then dust them with coconut shreds or chopped nuts. Freeze until firm for a delicious and portion-controlled dessert that's perfect for satisfying late-night cravings.
- Incorporating these bariatric-friendly recipes into your meal plan can help support your weight loss journey while still enjoying delicious and satisfying meals and snacks. Remember to listen to your body's signals of hunger and fullness and make adjustments as needed to fit your individual needs and preferences.

CHAPTER FIVE

5. Special Dietary Considerations

When it comes to food, there's a wide spectrum of dietary needs and preferences. Understanding and accommodating these needs is essential for creating inclusive and enjoyable dining experiences for everyone. Whether it's due to health reasons, personal beliefs, or cultural practices, special dietary considerations play a significant role in menu planning and meal preparation.

One of the most common dietary considerations is vegetarianism. Vegetarians abstain from consuming meat, poultry, and seafood, but they may still eat dairy products and eggs. For many vegetarians, this dietary choice is rooted in ethical, environmental, or health-related concerns.

5.1 Vegetarian Options

Creating vegetarian options involves more than just omitting meat from a dish. It's about crafting flavorful and satisfying meals that are packed with nutrients and variety.

Plant-based proteins like beans, lentils, tofu, and tempeh can serve as excellent substitutes for meat in recipes. Incorporating a diverse array of vegetables, grains, nuts, and seeds not only adds depth to the dish but also ensures a well-rounded nutritional profile.

From hearty salads and vegetable stir-fries to indulgent pasta dishes and savory veggie burgers, the possibilities for vegetarian cuisine are endless. Experimenting with different spices, herbs, and cooking techniques can elevate vegetarian dishes to new heights, enticing even the most devout meat lovers.

5.2 Vegan Options

Veganism takes vegetarianism a step further by excluding all animal products, including dairy and eggs. For those following a vegan lifestyle, ethical considerations regarding animal welfare, environmental sustainability, and personal health are often the driving factors behind their dietary choices.
Crafting delicious vegan meals requires creativity and a willingness to explore alternative ingredients and cooking methods. Instead of relying on animal-derived products, chefs can harness the power of plant-based ingredients to create mouthwatering dishes that are both nutritious and satisfying.

5.3 Gluten-Free Recipes

Gluten is a protein found in wheat, barley, and rye, making it off-limits for individuals with celiac disease or gluten sensitivity. For these individuals, consuming gluten-containing foods can trigger a range of symptoms, from digestive issues to fatigue and joint pain. As a result, gluten-free diets have become increasingly popular, not only among those with gluten-related disorders but also among people seeking alternative dietary choices.

Fortunately, there's a growing variety of gluten-free ingredients and products available on the market, making it easier than ever to enjoy a diverse range of gluten-free recipes. From gluten-free flours made from rice, almond, or chickpeas to gluten-free pasta, bread, and baked goods, there's no shortage of options for those following a gluten-free lifestyle.

5.4 Dairy-Free Alternatives

For individuals who are lactose intolerant or have dairy allergies, finding suitable alternatives to milk, cheese, and other dairy products is essential. Fortunately, there's been a surge in dairy-free options in recent years, ranging from plant-based milks like almond, soy, coconut, and oat milk to dairy-free cheeses, yogurts, and ice creams.

In addition to being suitable for those with dairy allergies or intolerances, dairy-free alternatives are also popular among vegans and individuals looking to reduce their consumption of animal products. These alternatives offer a wide range of flavors and textures, making it easy to enjoy all your favorite dairy-based dishes without compromising on taste or quality.

5.5   Incorporating Special Dietary Considerations into Menus

When designing menus for restaurants, catering events, or meal plans, it's essential to consider the diverse dietary needs and preferences of your audience. By offering a variety of vegetarian, vegan, gluten-free, and dairy-free options, you can ensure that everyone can find something delicious to enjoy.

One approach is to clearly label menu items with special dietary considerations, making it easy for guests to identify suitable options at a glance. Providing detailed information about ingredients and preparation methods can also help customers make informed choices about their meals.

Additionally, training kitchen staff on food safety protocols and cross-contamination prevention is crucial when catering to special dietary needs.

By taking steps to prevent cross-contact between allergens and ensuring that special dietary requests are handled with care, you can create a welcoming and inclusive dining experience for all.

Ultimately, special dietary considerations play a significant role in modern dining experiences, reflecting a growing awareness of diverse dietary needs and preferences. By offering a variety of vegetarian, vegan, gluten-free, and dairy-free options, chefs and foodservice professionals can create inclusive menus that cater to everyone, regardless of their dietary restrictions or preferences. With creativity, innovation, and a commitment to excellence, it's possible to create delicious and satisfying meals that delight customers of all backgrounds.

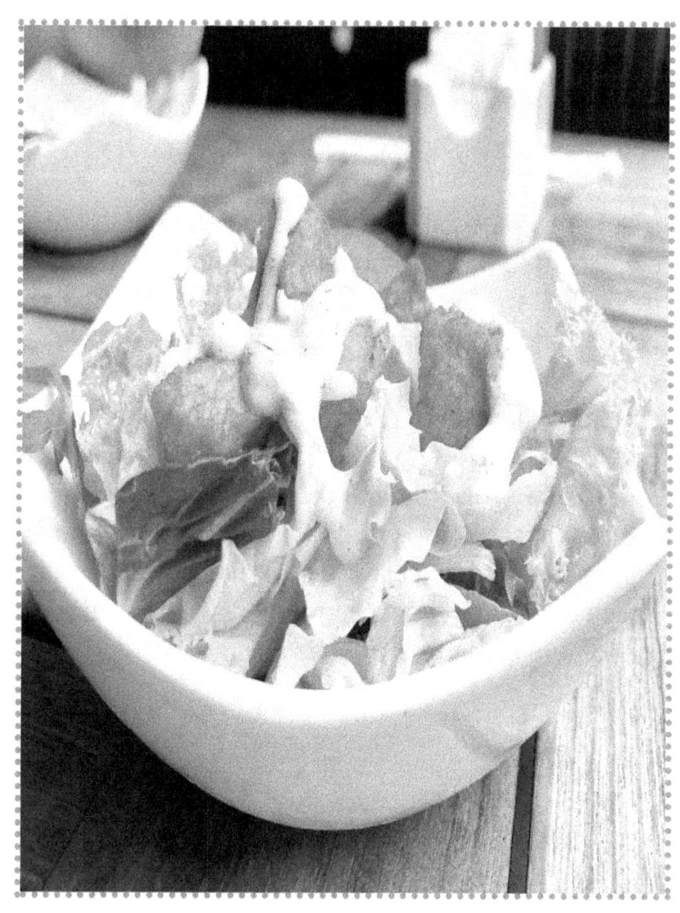

CHAPTER SIX

6. Nutritional Information and Tips under Bariatric Cooking

When it comes to bariatric cooking, nutrition is key. Bariatric surgery is a life-changing procedure that requires careful attention to diet and lifestyle. Whether you've undergone gastric bypass, sleeve gastrectomy, or another form of bariatric surgery, it's essential to prioritize nutrient-dense foods to support your health and weight loss goals.

6.1 Importance of Protein

Protein plays a crucial role in bariatric cooking and post-surgery recovery. After bariatric surgery, your body needs extra protein to support tissue repair, muscle growth, and metabolism. Aim to include protein-rich foods in every meal to promote satiety and prevent muscle loss. Good sources of protein include lean meats, poultry, fish, eggs, tofu, legumes, and dairy products. Incorporating protein supplements or shakes can also help you meet your protein needs, especially during the early stages of recovery when solid foods may be limited.

6.2 Essential Vitamins and Minerals

Supplementation is crucial because bariatric surgery may affect your body's capacity to absorb specific vitamins and minerals. Key nutrients to focus on include:

- **Vitamin B12**: Important for nerve function and red blood cell production. Bariatric patients often require lifelong B12 supplementation due to decreased absorption.

- **Iron**: Necessary for oxygen transport and energy production. Iron deficiency is common after bariatric surgery, so regular monitoring and supplementation may be needed.

- **Calcium**: Vital for bone health. Bariatric patients may have difficulty absorbing calcium, so calcium citrate supplements are often recommended.

- **Vitamin D**: Promotes immune system function and bone health. Many bariatric patients are deficient in vitamin D, so supplementation is typically advised.

- **Folate**: Essential for cell growth and DNA synthesis. Bariatric surgery can increase the risk of folate deficiency, so supplementation may be necessary.

In addition to supplements, focus on consuming nutrient-dense foods such as fruits, vegetables, whole grains, and fortified foods to meet your nutritional needs.

6.3 Hydration Guidelines

Staying hydrated is crucial for overall health and well-being, especially after bariatric surgery. Adequate hydration supports digestion, metabolism, and nutrient absorption, while also helping to prevent complications such as kidney stones and constipation. Here are some hydration guidelines to keep in mind:

1. **Drink plenty of water**: Aim to drink at least 64 ounces of water per day, sipping slowly throughout the day to avoid overwhelming your stomach.

2. **Limit caffeine and carbonation**: Beverages containing caffeine or carbonation can irritate the stomach lining and may contribute to dehydration. Opt for decaffeinated beverages and avoid carbonated drinks.

3. **Choose hydrating foods**: In addition to drinking fluids, incorporate hydrating foods such as fruits and vegetables into your diet. Foods with high water content, such as cucumbers, watermelon, and citrus fruits, can help you stay hydrated.

4. **Monitor urine color**: Aim for pale yellow urine, which indicates adequate hydration. Dark yellow urine may indicate dehydration, so drink more fluids if your urine is dark in color.

5. **Avoid sugary drinks**: Beverages high in sugar can contribute to weight gain and may not provide adequate hydration. Remain with water, herbal tea, and other calorie-conscious drinks.

By prioritizing protein, essential vitamins and minerals, and hydration in your bariatric cooking and lifestyle, you can support your health and weight loss journey post-surgery. Remember to work closely with your healthcare team to develop a personalized nutrition plan that meets your individual needs and goals. With dedication and mindful eating, you can achieve long-term success and improved quality of life after bariatric surgery.

CHAPTER SEVEN

7. Lifestyle Changes for Bariatric Patients

Bariatric surgery is a life-changing decision that requires significant adjustments to your lifestyle. It's not just about the surgery itself; it's about embracing a new way of living to support your health and weight loss goals. Here are some key lifestyle changes to consider post-bariatric surgery:

1. **Dietary Modifications**: After bariatric surgery, your stomach size is reduced, which means you'll need to adjust your eating habits accordingly. Focus on consuming smaller, nutrient-dense meals that are high in protein and low in refined sugars and fats. Avoid carbonated beverages and prioritize hydration with water.

2. **Regular Exercise**: Incorporating exercise into your routine is crucial for maintaining weight loss and improving overall health. Start with low-impact activities like walking or swimming, and gradually increase intensity as you build strength and endurance. On most days of the week, try to get in at least 30 minutes of moderate exercise.

3. **Behavioral Changes**: Bariatric surgery is not a quick fix; it requires a commitment to long-term behavioral changes. Practice mindful eating, listen to your body's hunger and fullness cues, and avoid emotional eating triggers. Seek support from a therapist or counselor if you struggle with disordered eating patterns.

4. **Vitamin and Mineral Supplementation**: Bariatric surgery can impact your body's ability to absorb certain nutrients, so it's essential to take prescribed vitamin and mineral supplements to prevent deficiencies. Work closely with your healthcare team to determine the appropriate supplements for your needs.

7.1 Support for Bariatric Patients

Embarking on a bariatric journey can feel overwhelming, but you don't have to go it alone. Building a strong support network can provide encouragement, accountability, and valuable resources along the way. Here's how to cultivate a supportive environment:

1. **Join a Support Group**: Connecting with others who have undergone bariatric surgery can be incredibly empowering. Look for local support groups or online communities where you can share experiences, ask questions, and receive

encouragement from people who understand what you're going through.

2. **Involve Your Loved Ones**: Share your journey with friends and family members and let them know how they can support you. Whether it's preparing healthy meals together, joining you for walks, or simply offering words of encouragement, having the support of loved ones can make a significant difference.

3. **Work with a Healthcare Team**: Your healthcare team, including your surgeon, dietitian, and mental health professional, are invaluable resources for guidance and support. Attend follow-up appointments regularly, ask questions, and don't hesitate to reach out if you need assistance navigating challenges.

4. **Practice Self-Compassion**: Be patient and kind to yourself throughout the bariatric journey. Celebrate your successes, no matter how small, and forgive yourself for setbacks. Remember that progress is not always linear, and it's okay to ask for help when you need it.

7.2 Incorporating Exercise into Your Routine

Exercise plays a critical role in maintaining weight loss, improving physical fitness, and enhancing overall well-being. Here are some tips for incorporating exercise into your routine post-bariatric surgery:

1. **Start Slow**: If you're new to exercise or recovering from surgery, start with gentle activities like walking or yoga. As your strength and endurance improve, gradually increase the duration and intensity of your workouts.

2. **Find Things You Love to Do**: Working out doesn't have to be a chore. Choose activities that you genuinely enjoy, whether it's dancing, cycling, swimming, or hiking. When you find something you love, you're more likely to stick with it long term.

3. **Schedule Regular Workouts**: Treat exercise like any other appointment and schedule it into your day. Aim for consistency by setting aside time for physical activity most days of the week. Remember that even short bursts of exercise can add up over time.

4. **Mix It Up**: Keep your workouts interesting by incorporating a variety of activities and exercises. Try different cardio workouts, strength training

routines, and flexibility exercises to challenge your body and prevent boredom.

7.3 Building a Support Network

Steering the challenges of weight loss and bariatric surgery is easier when you have a strong support network by your side. The following are some methods for creating a community that is encouraging:

1. **Reach Out to Others**: Don't be afraid to reach out to friends, family members, or fellow bariatric patients for support. Sharing your experiences and challenges with others who understand can provide comfort and encouragement.

2. **Join Support Groups**: Look for local support groups or online communities for bariatric patients. These groups often provide a safe space to ask questions, share advice, and celebrate successes with others who are on a similar journey.

3. **Attend Follow-Up Appointments**: Stay connected with your healthcare team by attending follow-up appointments regularly. These appointments provide an opportunity to address any concerns, track your progress, and receive

guidance on nutrition, exercise, and overall wellness.

4. **Consider Professional Support**: If you're struggling with emotional eating, body image issues, or other mental health concerns, consider seeking support from a therapist or counselor who specializes in bariatric surgery and weight management.

7.4 Coping with Emotional Eating

Emotional eating can be a significant challenge for bariatric patients, but there are strategies you can use to cope effectively. Here's how to manage emotional eating:

1. **Identify Triggers**: Pay attention to the situations, emotions, or thoughts that trigger emotional eating episodes. Common triggers include stress, boredom, sadness, loneliness, and anxiety. Once you identify your triggers, you can develop healthier coping mechanisms to manage them.

2. **Practice Mindful Eating**: Cultivate awareness and mindfulness around your eating habits. Pay attention to physical hunger and fullness cues, and eat slowly and mindfully without distractions. Engage all your senses and savor each bite of food.

3. **Find Alternative Coping Strategies**: Instead of turning to food for comfort, explore alternative coping strategies that soothe your emotions without sabotaging your health goals. Try deep breathing exercises, meditation, journaling, spending time in nature, or engaging in hobbies you enjoy.

4. 4. **Seek Support**: If you're having trouble with emotional eating, don't be afraid to ask friends, family, or mental health professionals for help.. Talking about your feelings and receiving validation and support can help you break free from unhealthy patterns.

Finally, bariatric surgery is just the beginning of a lifelong journey toward improved health and well-being. By making positive lifestyle changes, building a strong support network, incorporating exercise into your routine, and learning to cope with emotional eating, you can maximize the benefits of bariatric surgery and achieve long-term success. Remember to be patient with yourself, celebrate your progress, and seek help when you need it. You're not alone on this journey, and with dedication and support, you can achieve your goals and live a healthier, happier life.

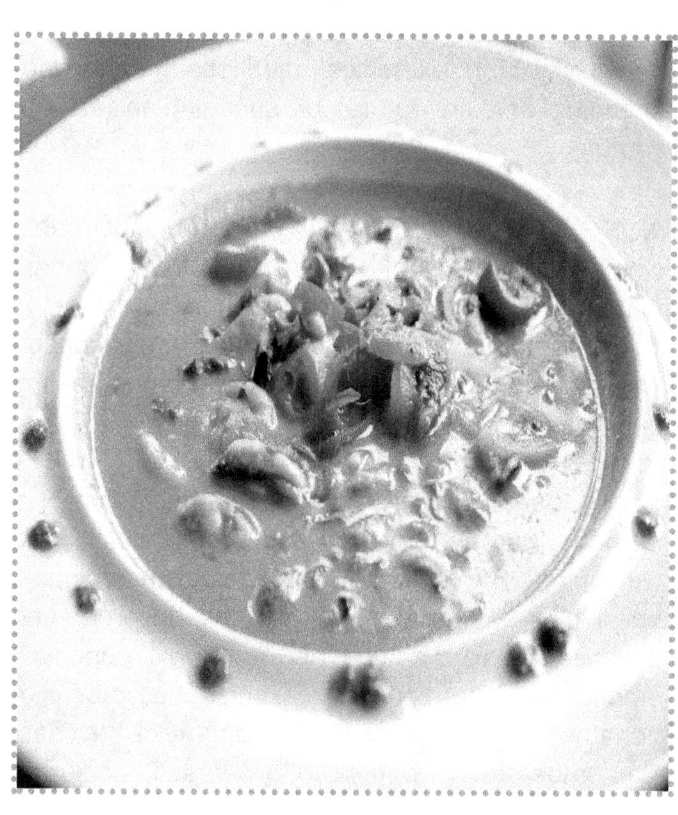

CHAPTER EIGHT

8. Frequently Asked Questions (FAQs) about the Bariatric Diet

- **What is a Bariatric Diet?**

  A Bariatric Diet is a specialized eating plan designed for individuals who have undergone bariatric surgery, such as gastric bypass or sleeve gastrectomy. It focuses on promoting weight loss and ensuring proper nutrition while accommodating the changes in the digestive system post-surgery.

- **Why is the Bariatric Diet necessary?**

  After bariatric surgery, the stomach's size is reduced, which limits the amount of food it can hold. Additionally, the surgery alters the digestive process, affecting how nutrients are absorbed. Therefore, following a specific diet is crucial for maximizing weight loss, preventing complications, and maintaining overall health.

- **What are the main principles of the Bariatric Diet?**

The Bariatric Diet typically involves:

1. **High Protein Intake:** Protein is essential for preserving muscle mass and promoting satiety.

2. **Low Carbohydrate Consumption:** Limiting carbs helps control blood sugar levels and aids in weight loss.

3. **Moderate Fat Intake:** Choosing healthy fats in moderation supports nutrient absorption and provides energy.

4. **Emphasis on Nutrient-Dense Foods:** Prioritizing foods rich in vitamins, minerals, and fiber helps meet nutritional needs despite consuming fewer calories.

5. **Small, Frequent Meals:** Eating smaller portions throughout the day prevents overeating and supports digestion.

- **What foods should be included in the Bariatric Diet?**

- The Bariatric Diet should consist of:

- Lean proteins from foods like tofu, fish, poultry, and eggs.

- Non-starchy vegetables like spinach, broccoli, and peppers.

- Whole grains in moderation, such as quinoa, brown rice, and oats.

- Low-fat dairy products or dairy alternatives.

- Healthy fats from sources like avocados, nuts, and olive oil.

- Limited amounts of fruits, focusing on those lower in sugar such as berries.

- **How does the Bariatric Diet differ from other weight loss diets?**

Unlike traditional weight loss diets, the Bariatric Diet is tailored to accommodate the changes in the digestive system post-surgery. It prioritizes high protein intake to preserve muscle mass, limits carbohydrates to aid in weight loss and blood sugar control, and emphasizes nutrient-dense foods to prevent nutrient deficiencies despite consuming fewer calories.

- **Is exercise important while following the Bariatric Diet?**

Yes, incorporating regular exercise into your routine is crucial for achieving and maintaining weight loss, improving overall health, and enhancing mood and energy levels. However, it's essential to consult with your healthcare provider before starting any exercise program to ensure it's safe and appropriate for your individual needs.

- **How can I prevent nutritional deficiencies on the Bariatric Diet?**

To prevent nutritional deficiencies, it's important to:

- Follow your healthcare provider's recommended supplement regimen, which typically includes vitamins and minerals such as calcium, vitamin D, vitamin B12, and iron.

- Choose nutrient-dense foods and focus on variety to ensure you're getting a wide range of essential nutrients.

- Monitor your nutrient levels regularly through blood tests and consult with your healthcare provider if you have any concerns or symptoms of deficiency.

8.1 Common Concerns About the Bariatric Diet

Will I feel hungry on the Bariatric Diet?

It's normal to experience hunger sensations, especially in the initial stages of adjusting to the Bariatric Diet. However, focusing on high-protein foods and smaller, more frequent meals can help manage hunger and promote feelings of fullness. Drinking water between meals can also help curb hunger.

What are some common challenges of the Bariatric Diet?

Some common challenges of the Bariatric Diet include:

- Adapting to smaller portion sizes and limited food choices.

- Dealing with food cravings and emotional eating habits.

- Ensuring adequate hydration, as the reduced stomach size may impact fluid intake.

- Managing social situations and dining out while adhering to dietary restrictions.

How can I stop emotional eating and food cravings?

In order to stop emotional eating and food cravings, it can be useful to:

- Identify triggers and develop coping strategies such as practicing mindfulness, engaging in stress-relieving activities, or seeking support from a therapist or support group.

- Focus on satisfying nutrient-rich foods that promote satiety and provide long-lasting energy.

- Practice mindful eating by paying attention to hunger and fullness cues and savoring each bite.

What should I do if I experience digestive issues on the Bariatric Diet?

If you experience digestive issues such as nausea, vomiting, or diarrhea, it's essential to:

- Slow down when eating and chew food thoroughly to aid digestion.

- Avoid carbonated beverages, high-fat foods, and foods that are difficult to digest.

- Stay hydrated and sip fluids between meals rather than with meals.

- Consult with your healthcare provider if digestive issues persist or worsen.

8.2   Tips for Dining Out on the Bariatric Diet

What are some healthier options I can choose when eating out?

When dining out on the Bariatric Diet, consider the following tips:

- Review the menu beforehand and look for protein-rich options such as grilled chicken, fish, or lean cuts of meat.

- Instead of frying, choose foods that are baked, grilled, or steamed.

- Request modifications such as substituting side dishes for vegetables or asking for sauces and dressings on the side.

- Pay attention to portion sizes and think about splitting a meal or putting half away for later.

- Limit alcoholic beverages, sugary drinks, and high-calorie desserts.

What are some strategies for navigating social situations involving food?

8.3 Steering social situations involving food can be challenging, but these strategies can help:

- Communicate your dietary needs and restrictions to friends and family members in advance.

- Offer to bring a dish or suggest restaurants with options that align with your dietary preferences.

- Focus on socializing and enjoying the company of others rather than solely on food.

- Practice assertiveness and politely decline foods that don't align with your dietary goals.

How can I manage cravings and temptations while dining out?

8.4 To manage cravings and temptations while dining out:

- Plan ahead by eating a small, protein-rich snack before heading to the restaurant to curb hunger and reduce the likelihood of overeating.

- Choose a restaurant with healthier options or ask if the chef can accommodate your dietary needs.

- Practice mindful eating by paying attention to hunger and fullness cues and savoring each bite.

- Remind yourself of your goals and the reasons why you're following the Bariatric Diet to stay motivated and focused.

8.5 Managing Plateaus and Setbacks on the Bariatric Diet

How do I proceed if I reach a weight loss plateau?

If you hit a weight loss plateau on the Bariatric Diet, consider the following strategies:

- Evaluate your diet and exercise routine to identify any areas where you can make improvements or changes.

- Mix up your exercise routine by trying new activities or increasing the intensity or duration of your workouts.

- Focus on non-scale victories such as improvements in energy levels, fitness, and overall health rather than solely on the number on the scale.

- Stay patient and consistent with your efforts, as weight loss plateaus are common and often temporary.

8.6   How can I stay motivated during setbacks or challenges?

Staying motivated during setbacks or challenges on the Bariatric Diet can be tough, but these tips can help:

- Focus on your reasons for undergoing bariatric surgery and the positive changes you've experienced since then.

- Set realistic goals and

CHAPTER NINE

9. Conclusion

Congratulations! You've kick-start on a transformative journey towards better health and well-being through bariatric surgery. This decision marks a significant turning point in your life, one that requires commitment, dedication, and resilience. As you reflect on your experiences leading up to this moment, it's important to acknowledge the courage it took to take this step towards a healthier future.

Your bariatric journey is not just about physical transformation; it's also a journey of self-discovery and empowerment. Along the way, you've likely faced challenges and obstacles, but you've also discovered inner strength and resilience you may not have known you possessed. Embrace this journey as an opportunity for growth and personal development, knowing that every step forward brings you closer to your goals.

As you move forward post-surgery, remember that the road to long-term success is paved with consistent effort and mindful choices. While bariatric surgery is a powerful tool for weight loss, it's not a quick fix. It requires a commitment to making sustainable lifestyle changes, including adopting a healthy diet, staying physically active, and prioritizing self-care.

9.1   Final Thoughts on Your Bariatric Journey

Your bariatric journey is a testament to your courage and determination to live a healthier, happier life. It's a journey that is uniquely yours, filled with ups and downs, triumphs and setbacks. As you navigate the challenges and celebrate the victories, remember to be kind to yourself and practice self-compassion.

One of the most important aspects of your bariatric journey is building a strong support system. Surround yourself with people who uplift and encourage you, whether it's friends, family, or fellow bariatric patients. Lean on them for support during difficult times, and celebrate your successes together.

Additionally, don't hesitate to seek professional guidance when needed. Your bariatric team, including surgeons, dietitians, and mental health professionals, are here to support you every step of the way. Be open and honest with them about your struggles and concerns, and trust their expertise to help you overcome obstacles and achieve your goals.

Above all, remember that your bariatric journey is a marathon, not a sprint. Remain persistent and patient, and have faith in the process. Celebrate your progress, no matter how small, and keep your eyes focused on the bright future that awaits you.

9.2 Supportive Resources

1. **Online Communities**

- BariatricPal: An online community for bariatric patients to connect, share experiences, and support each other through their journeys.

- ObesityHelp: A comprehensive resource for individuals considering or undergoing bariatric surgery, offering forums, articles, and educational materials.

2. **Nutrition and Meal Planning**

- MyFitnessPal: A popular app for tracking food intake, exercise, and weight loss progress. It offers a vast database of foods and recipes to help you stay on track with your nutrition goals.

- Bariatric Foodie: A website dedicated to providing bariatric-friendly recipes, meal plans, and tips for successful post-op eating.

3. **Fitness and Exercise**

- Fitbit: A wearable fitness tracker that monitors your activity levels, heart rate, and sleep patterns. It provides motivation and accountability to help you stay active and reach your fitness goals.

- Daily Burn: An online platform offering a variety of workout programs, including cardio, strength training, yoga, and more. With on-demand workouts led by certified trainers, you can exercise anytime, anywhere.

4. **Mental Health and Support**

- Talkspace: An online therapy platform that connects you with licensed therapists for virtual counseling sessions. It's a convenient and accessible option for addressing mental health concerns and receiving support during your bariatric journey.

- Obesity Action Coalition (OAC): A non-profit organization dedicated to advocating for individuals affected by obesity. The OAC offers support groups, educational resources, and advocacy initiatives to empower individuals on their weight loss journeys.

Remember, you're not alone on this journey. With the right support, resources, and mindset, you can achieve your goals and live the healthy, fulfilling life you deserve. Keep pushing forward, and never lose sight of the incredible progress you've already made. Your best days are still ahead of you!

9.3 DAILY MEAL REMAKE

>Daily Meal Remake<

S/N	DAILY	MEAL	REMAKE

			58
